ENERGY MISMATCH:

HORMONES, ENZYMES, VIRUSES, HEAVY METALS, VACCINATIONS, DRUGS, ALLERGENS, FLOWER REMEDIES, HOMEOPATHICS & MORE

Jane Thurnell-Read

Previously published as ISBN: 0954243935 (2004)

ISBN: 978-0-9542439-3-7

Published by:

Life-Work Potential
Sea View House
Long Rock
Penzance
Cornwall
TR20 8JF
England

Tel: +44 (0)1736 719030
www.lifeworkpotential.com

Other books by the author:

Health Kinesiology: The Muscle Testing System That Talks To The Body, ISBN: 9780954243968, Life-Work Potential Limited, 2009

The Guide To Geopathic Stress, ISBN 1 84333 529 8, Vega, 2002 (out of print)

Geopathic Stress & Subtle Energy, ISBN: 0954243943, Life-Work Potential Limited, 2006

Verbal Questioning Skills For Kinesiologists, ISBN: 9780954243913, Life-Work Potential Limited, 2002

Allergy A To Z, ISBN: 0954243927, Life-Work Potential Limited 2005

Nutritional Testing For Kinesiologists And Dowsers, ISBN 9780954243951, Life-Work Potential Limited, 2009

Visit www.healthandgodness.com for tips, information and inspiration for a happier, healthier life.

Visit www.mytherapypractice.com for articles and information for students and practitioners of alternative and complementary medicine.

Visit our online shop at www.lifeworkpotential.com for test kits, books, etc.

Contents

The basic procedures shown here are taken from
Health Kinesiology (HK)
developed by
Jimmy Scott, Ph.D.

Jane Thurnell-Read has been a kinesiology practitioner for over 20 years. She has written numerous articles, been interviewed on radio and television, and had several books published.

During this time she has helped thousands of people with a wide range of problems. She considers that the energy mismatch concept is one of the most important factors in her high success rate with clients.

One of her biggest contributions to work in this field has been the development of a comprehensive range of test kits, backed up by extensive research and detailed information for the practitioner. This enables practitioners to take full advantage of the power of the energy mismatch concept.

At one time she taught the material as a one-day workshop, but she has now retired from teaching and seeing clients in order to concentrate on writing and research. There is a continuing demand for this information, so she decided to write this book.

How To Use This Book

Depending on your skills and experience you can use this book in different ways:

1. If you a kinesiologist or TFH'er, you will want to read this book in full and use the protocol as it is described.

2. If you are trained in health kinesiology, you may prefer to use the symbiotic energy transformation (SET) technique instead of the tapping technique, providing the energy system gives you permission to do so.

3. If you use an EAV, Vega or Biocom machine or something similar, you may want to use your normal diagnostic procedures, but still read the information on pages 4 to 6, so that you get a thorough grounding in the concept of energy mismatch. Having used your existing skills to work out the problem items, you can then use the correcting procedures taught here to rectify the situation.

A summary of the full protocol is set out on page 77.

What Is Energy Mismatch?

In our normal lives we encounter many different substances: food, personal care products, household cleaners, things we inhale or touch, drugs and supplements, viruses, bacteria, fungi, and possibly even parasites. The body has to decide how to react to any of these physical substances it encounters. This is a critical process, because it determines the processes that are put in train by the body, and what happens to the substance.

For example, if the body considers a substance in the mouth to be something it wants, it will produce digestive juices, etc., in order to maximise absorption. On the other hand if the ingested substance is viewed as harmful, vomiting or diarrhoea may occur. If something entering the nose is viewed as beneficial, the airways open and breathing becomes deeper to allow easy entry, but if it is categorised as harmful, narrowing of the air passages or copious production of mucus may result, in order to block or hinder entry.

Sometimes, however, the body / energy system seems to mis-categorise something, and this can have serious implications for health.

There are three basic possibilities:

1. Something beneficial is miscategorised as harmful
2. Something harmful is miscategorised as beneficial
3. Something is uncategorised

If the body categorises something harmful as beneficial, it will do its best to enhance absorption of the substance, even though it is harmful. If it categorises something beneficial as harmful, it will do its best to block entry, and failing that to excrete the substance as quickly as possible from the body, minimising absorption. If it is unable to categorise it at all, it will not know what to do with it. All of these situations can lead to all sorts of health problems.

The body also has to categorise and react appropriately to substances produced within the body itself. In many ways the body can be seen as a complex chemical factory, producing a wide range of chemicals. Some chemicals are used where they are produced. Some are produced in one area, but travel around the body either continuously in the blood stream or to target another organ. The body also produces waste products (e.g. ammonia, urea) as a result of all this chemical activity. These need to be either recycled or excreted.

Efficient functioning at this level of complexity is in part dependent on the body recognising the substance appropriately. If it does not recognise a useful substance for what it is, it may try to break it down or excrete it from the body. A metabolic by-product may be stored rather than excreted. These and other problems can result in a whole range of health problems.

The energy mismatch test determines whether or not the energy system recognises the substances appropriately. It checks if the energy system will attempt to use the substance appropriately.

Both the testing procedure and the correcting procedure are very simple, but the results can be dramatic, across a wide range of different complaints.

Here are some comments from kinesiologists who have used this technique very successfully:

> "I have had fantastic results with the energy mismatch, particularly with blood sugar problems and hormone problems."

> "I had brilliant results with energy mismatch on a fellow kinesiologist's horse, who was covered in large hot lumps and had lost all his zest for life. The vet was defeated by it.... The problem turned out to be an ingredient in his feed. For a day or two after the treatment the lumps got hotter and worse and then vanished. He is now a bouncing happy horse as his spirits returned as well."

The energy mismatch concept is one of the most useful I know: it has broad applications, and the testing and correcting procedures are very simple, and yet the results can be extraordinary.

Balancing The Meridian Energy System

Before checking anything we need to ensure that the client's energy system is balanced. This will mean that answers to our testing are likely to be accurate. Different kinesiologies have different ways of doing this.

In general most people will come in with an unbalanced energy system, and the health kinesiology thymus tap is a quick way to balance the energy system. This works for most people most of the time.

Either the therapist or the client can tap over the thymus area of the client. On an adult this is about 2 inches (5 cms) below the "v" where the breastbone and the collar bone meet. The tapping should be in a counter-clockwise circle, 3 inches (7.5 cms) in diameter. Tap with one or two fingers for about 30 seconds.

Some people find the concept of counter-clockwise difficult to understand in this context, but think of it as 'up from the heart'. The heart is on the left side of the body, so you start on the upper chest on the left side (as the client would name it), tap upwards and over in a circle.

I do not find it matters how many fingers I use when I do this tapping. In general I use three, simply because that is physically what I do naturally. I know some kinesiologists are concerned about finger polarity. If you are one of these, it is a simple matter to tap with two fingers only. Some clients feel that they are being ‘poked’ if you only use one finger, so I do not advise this.

Checking That The Meridian Energy System Is Balanced

The thymus tap is usually sufficient to balance the energy system. It is important not to assume that is the case, but to run some checks. Different kinesiologies have different pre-checks. Because I only use HK procedures in my practice, I do not know if others are adequate for checking for balance before proceeding with the energy mismatch protocol. The HK pre-checks test different aspects of energy balance. I suggest that when you first work with the energy mismatch protocol you carry out these checks either instead of or in addition to any normal pre-checks you would use.

During this protocol you will be doing a lot of testing, so it is important to find a convenient muscle to use. I usually use the brachioradialis (in the lower forearm) if possible. This is because it is easy to explain to the client what you want them to do. When the client is lying down the lower arm rests on the couch / bench, with the forearm at ninety degrees to the couch. The thumb should be pointing towards the head and the palm facing inwards. Light pressure is applied just below the wrist. The full range of movement takes the arm down to the couch. If this muscle is not suitable for some reason (through injury or because it does not test strong in the clear), I might use the anterior deltoid or the latissimus dorsi instead. It is also possible to carry out this protocol using self-testing or surrogate testing. In which case you would need to adapt the instructions accordingly.

It is important that the energy system 'passes' all these checks. If it does not, you stop at the first failure, repeat the tapping procedure on page 7, and then carry out the checks again. If the energy system still fails these pre-checks, you will need to use other techniques to balance the body, and then recheck.

The steps are:

1. Find a muscle that tests strong in the clear.
2. With palm of the hand over the navel, test any muscle in the clear. It should lock (test strong) if the person is balanced.
3. With palm over the navel, pinch in the belly (the middle) of any muscle and test a different muscle. It should unlock (test weak) if the person is balanced. The pinch should be longitudinal towards the centre of the muscle.
4. With palm over the navel, unpinch in the belly of the same muscle and test an indicator muscle. This time you smooth outwards towards the end of the muscle. The muscle should lock if the person is balanced. If it does not lock, the reason is usually because you have not 'unpinched' the muscle sufficiently. To unpinch a muscle smooth the fibres back together, going in the opposite direction to the pinching.
5. With palm over the navel, test the indicator muscle, as the client says "no". It should unlock if the person is balanced.
6. With palm over the navel, test the indicator muscle, as the client says "yes". It should lock if the person is balanced.

7. With palm over the navel, place the north-seeking pole of a magnet on the belly of any muscle and test the indicator muscle. It should unlock if the person is balanced. The magnets many people are familiar with have the poles at the end. These can be used, but it is a bit precarious to balance the magnet on its end. I use a magnet that has been axially magnetised. This means that the pole is along the flat face of the magnet, so it is much more convenient.
8. With palm over the navel, place the south-seeking pole of a magnet on the belly of any muscle and test the indicator muscle. It should lock if the person is balanced.

Remember that it is important that the energy system 'passes' all these checks. The magnet test is particularly useful, because it is possible to do it blind or even double blind. With the pinch test and the yes/no test clients are aware of what you are doing. Experienced clients will often know what the 'correct' response is and so try to be helpful and allow their arm to test weak at the appropriate point. However, for the magnet test, they do not know which way the magnet is facing (unless you always do the test in the same order), and so do not know what the 'correct' response is. You can make this an even more profound test, by checking the magnet without you or the client knowing which pole is against the body.

Occasionally you will find people who 'pass' on all the other tests, but fail the magnet test. If this happens, try getting them to drink water, and then retest. If this still fails, it is likely that the magnet is disturbing their energy system: the client is balanced, but becomes unbalanced as soon as you put the magnet in their energy field. If a client's own electro-magnetic integrity is not robust, they will often go out of balance immediately a magnet is put near them. These people are often also very sensitive to electro-magnetic pollution and geopathic stress, and will suffer from static electric shocks. If this is the case, they almost certainly need degaussing (see page 79), so do this and then carry out the magnet tests again.

These three tests (pinching, yes/no and magnet) are checking different aspects of energy balance and all need to be correct. If you get the reverse response from any of the tests, tap the thymus again and re-check.

For steps 2-8 a hand needs to be over the client's navel. It can be the person's hand, the therapist's hand or a third person's hand. In practice I usually use my hand, because by the time I have explained to the client what I want them to do, I could have completed the test if I put my hand over the client's navel. By putting the palm of the hand over the navel in this way, you are covering a combination of points that connect in to all the meridians, so this test allows you to check that all the meridians are in balance without needing to check a muscle connected with each one individually.

I usually pinch the quadriceps muscle, as this is a convenient muscle to use while the client is lying or sitting down. If the indicator muscle does not unlock, this could be because you have not pinched hard enough. If you suspect this, try pinching again. It is important when you pinch the muscle that you really do pinch the physical muscle, because you are definitely testing something about the physiological response of the body, involving the spindle cells in the belly of the muscle. Pinching just off the body or extremely lightly does not affect the muscle fibres, so is not appropriate. To pinch a muscle you must pinch along the fibres of the muscle. In the case of the quadriceps this means pinching along the leg, not across it. In pinching we are checking that a physiological response from one muscle can be picked up by the indicator muscle.

Testing For Energy Mismatch

Now that the person is balanced, you can start checking whether or not the energy system recognises something correctly – the energy mismatch test.

This test works regardless of whether the substance being tested is a beneficial substance or a harmful substance. It simply means that the energy system has got the substance wrongly labelled, or is unable to label it at all.

The hand is <u>not</u> on the navel when performing the following energy mismatch tests, because we are now using a specific test point.

The energy mismatch test point is located at triple warmer 21 (TW21). Triple warmer 21 is in front of the ear. Fortunately it is not necessary to touch the spot precisely. By laying your finger or the client's finger in front of the ear you will cover the point. If you are concerned about finger polarity, use two fingers. Remove the finger from in front of the ear between tests to avoid 'fatiguing' the test point.

First you need to test TW21 in the clear. Very occasionally it will test weak in the clear. In this case you should tap both TW21's and both Lung 5's (just above the crook of the elbow, on the side closest to the thumb). You can tap these in any order. Retest TW21 in the clear, and it should now test strong.

The substance being tested is placed on central or conception vessel 6 (CV6). This is situated approximately two finger widths (the client's) below the navel on the midline. For most people it is perfectly acceptable to test the substance through clothing or in a container, but see appendix 2 for some restrictions. You test the indicator muscle while the substance is on CV6 and one TW21 is held.

For this test you can use actual substances (e.g. an apple, hair from the client's dog, etc.), or you can use test kits, which contain radionics or homeopathic energy patterns of the substances. To maximise your accuracy only test one thing at a time.

Here is a summary of the actual testing procedure:

1. Without the hand on the navel, test one TW21 in the clear. It will normally test strong.
2. If it tests weak, tap *both* TW21's and *both* Lung 5's - just above the crook of the elbows, and then retest.
3. Place the sample or test kit vial you want to test on CV6, hold TW21 and test an indicator muscle.
4. If the indicator muscle tests weak, this means that the body does not recognise the energy pattern of the substance correctly. If the indicator tests strong, this means that the energy system does recognise the energy pattern of the substance correctly.

It is possible quickly to test a whole range of substances. In practice you are likely to want to test and then correct any mismatched substance as you go along. See page 73 for information on deciding what to test.

People can have problems with a substance for other reasons. If this is the case, it will not show up through this testing procedure. For example, if the client has a low tolerance (as opposed to an allergy) to the test substance, this will not show up on the energy mismatch point. Similarly if the person is experiencing unpleasant reactions to something because it is toxic, this will not show up either.

Sometimes the body is reacting physically to a substance, often where membranes are already inflamed. Typical examples of this are where people react to strong perfumes or cigarette smoke, because these irritate the mucus membranes in their nose, which are already inflamed for other reasons. Someone with colitis may react to wholemeal bread because the bran in it is physically 'scrubbing' the tender membranes in the colon. This type of reaction will not show up on the energy mismatch point either, unless the person is actually allergic to the substance.

Correcting Energy Mismatch Problems

You may have procedures within your own kinesiology that will allow you to correct energy mismatch problems, but I urge you to try this way if you are not already familiar with it. It has been used by many different students and practitioners with outstanding results. It is a very robust way of correcting problems. In general it does not need to be repeated: once it is fixed it usually stays fixed. Once again it is a procedure from HK.

Do remember that this is a procedure that only corrects energy mismatch problems, so it will not help if inflamed membranes cause the problem, for example. Also this is a correction for allergy problems, not for tolerance problems (see page 27).

The HK tapping technique will not always work, so first you need to find out if it will work for the substance you want to correct. The test point for this is Heart 1. Heart 1 is in the middle of the armpit. You need to hold both H1's. It is usually most convenient to get the client to hold one, and for you to hold the other one. During these tests you do not have a hand over the client's navel nor do you hold TW21, but the substance is on CV6.

This is how you check if the tapping procedure will work:

1. With the substance on CV6 hold both H1's in the client's armpits and test the indicator muscle. (Do not hold TW21)
2. If the arm tests weak, the tapping procedure will work. If the arm locks, the tapping procedure will not work.

If testing shows that the tapping technique will not work, you need to look for other alternatives. HK teaches a very powerful technique called the symbiotic energy transformation (SET) technique. This will usually work when the tapping technique will not.

Even when testing shows that the tapping will work, you still need to establish whether it is an appropriate thing to do for the client. Sometimes it is not appropriate. For example, when you have already corrected a lot of substances in the session, or when the person has had other heavy-duty energy work done either in the session or in the days before.

The easiest way to establish this is by asking the verbal question:

> 'Do we have energy permission to correct the energy mismatch problem for this substance right now?'

As you ask the question, apply light pressure on the indicator muscle. While you ask this question you do not have the substance on CV6, and you do not hold TW21.

A strong response means "yes". Do not proceed without this permission. If you continue, the person may experience extreme and unpleasant side effects of the treatment.

If you get 'no', it does not mean that you can never correct it, just that it is not appropriate to do it right now. In fact, it may be appropriate to correct that substance later in the session, after you have corrected one or more other substances, or done some other treatment. You can establish this by asking more verbal questions. (See my book *Verbal Questioning Skills For Kinesiologists* for more information.)

So, in order to proceed to the tapping you need to find a weak/unlocked response to the Heart 1 test, and a strong/locked response to the verbal question.

Once you know that the energy tapping will work (the Heart 1 test) and that it is appropriate to do it (the verbal question), you can continue with the procedure.

For this you need once again to put the substance back on CV6. Then you tap gently but firmly in any order the beginning and end points of the bladder, kidney, stomach and spleen meridians for about 20-30 seconds.

If you use one finger for your tapping, you need to be extremely precise. Normally I use two or three fingers; this allows me to tap quickly, but be confident that I am covering the correct spot.

The points can be tapped by you, the client or a third party. Usually I tap some and get the client to tap other points. If you are working on a surrogate, it still works if you tap the points on the surrogate, providing the surrogate is in physical contact with the client.

Here are the locations of the points:

Bladder 1:
Beside the nose at the inner corner of each eye

Bladder 67:
At the lateral corner of the base of the nails of the little toes (the lateral side is the side furthest away from the midline of the body)

Kidney 1:
Centre of the balls of the feet

Kidney 27:
Just below clavicle/sternum junction, either side of the sternum

Stomach 1:
On the eye socket bones just below the centre of the eyes

Stomach 45:
At the lateral corner of the base of the nails of the second toes (the toe next to the big toe, but the side furthest away from it)

Spleen 1:
At the medial corner of the base of the nails of the big toes (the side closest to the midline of the body)

Spleen 21:
The sides of the torso, straight down from the armpits, approximately level with the nipples

When you have finished tapping, you need to check that the correction is complete. With the substance still on CV6 hold TW21 and check that the indicator muscle now tests strong. If it does not, either tap all the points again, or use verbal questioning to establish which of the specific points need further tapping. When you have done this, you recheck as before.

I also recommend you check that the correction is complete by asking a verbal question. Remove the substance from CV6, and without holding TW21 ask:

> 'Is this completely and robustly done?'

A strong response means that it is robust. Occasionally you will get a strong response to the TW21 test and a 'no' to the verbal question. The main reason for this is because you have tapped the points long enough temporarily to change the energy system's response to the substance, but not long enough to give a really robust correction which will last over time, so you need to re-tap all or some of the points. With practice this situation is unlikely to occur.

Here is a summary of the correcting procedure:

1. With the substance on CV6 check that the correcting procedure will work (H1 test) – a weak response means the tap will work.
2. Without the substance on the body check that you have energy permission to correct the problem (verbal question) – a strong response means yes, you have permission.
3. Carry out the tap. (Only correct one substance at a time.)
4. With the substance on CV6 check that the correction is complete (TW21 test) – a strong response means it is.
5. Without the substance on the body, check that the correction is now robust (verbal question) – a strong response means it is.

The procedure itself is very simple. Once you have used it a few times you will find it quick and easy to do. The basic correcting procedure can be used in all sorts of situations. Most practitioners are amazed at the applications and implications of this simple testing and correcting procedure.

Using Actual Substances Versus Using Test Kits

In general you can use either actual substances or test vials for the test sample, but using the test vials have some big advantages in some circumstances:

1. Test vials allow you to have a large range of substances easily to hand. They occupy very little space and can be stored easily in boxes or bags ready for use.
2. Using the vials is ideal for people with severe allergies because you can carry out the whole procedure without physically exposing them to the substance.
3. Sometimes clients have strong (but wrong) views about what the problem substances are or are not. By using test vials, you can test things without the client trying to influence the result, as they are unable to tell what is being tested.
4. Using test vials also allows you, if you wish, to test things without you knowing what they are, so that your own preconceptions do not influence the result.
5. Many practitioners feel that using test vials enhances their professional image.
6. Some substances are too expensive in their normal physical form or are perishable, or just not readily available.

There are occasions when it is more appropriate to use the actual substance. For example, the client's own dog hair may test differently from a generalised dog hair testing vial. Drinking water varies geographically (because of the geology), by area (depending on the purification system used by that water authority) and between houses (depending on the materials used in the plumbing). The water used by your neighbour may not be exactly the same as yours, so when you test your neighbour use their water not your own.

Whether you are using real substances or test vials it is important to test one vial at a time, or simple rather than complex substances. So, it is not a good idea to test a kit, by putting the whole kit on CV6, nor is it a good idea to test a complex substance like bread or chocolate. Using simple substances and individual vials will enhance the accuracy of your testing, and the robustness of your correcting procedures.

There are several different manufacturers of test kits, but Life-Work Potential offer probably the largest range in the world, backed up with detailed information on the vials. (Contact details are in the front of this book.)

Waiting Before Re-Exposure

Correcting an allergy with the tapping technique corrects it immediately on an energy level, but it may be some time before this filters through to the physical body, so the person may be advised to avoid the substance(s) for a while. This can be anything from a few days to several months. The exact amount of time can be established through verbal questioning. However, it is not possible to avoid some things, so I generally advise clients to minimise their exposure as best they can. For example, if you have just fixed a house dust allergy, it is probably advisable for the client not to go home and do some dusting or vacuuming at least for several days.

If you have corrected an allergy to dental material that is in the client's mouth, it is impossible for them to avoid it, but nevertheless the client will still feel the benefit of the energy mismatch correction.

Tolerance

We all probably have tolerance levels for everything, but if your tolerance for oranges is 40 oranges a day, you are unlikely to be aware of any tolerance problems.

If you are allergic to something, your tolerance level is zero. Once the allergy is fixed, using the tapping technique or any other procedure, tolerance may rise gradually or immediately of its own accord.

Sometimes even though the allergy is fixed, tolerance levels do not rise sufficiently to be practically useful. For example, you might correct an allergy to oranges so that now the client can have 20 drops of orange juice a day. In practical terms this is still not going to allow the client to eat oranges. The client may return complaining that the tap did not work, because they still cannot eat oranges. Put an orange or a suitable test vial on CV6 and hold TW21 and re-check. If the arm tests strong, it means that they must still have low tolerance, and you will need to address this in another way. If the arm tests weak, it probably means that you did not tap for long enough initially and need to tap the points again.

Sometimes the client has never been allergic to a substance, but still has very low tolerance levels that will need working on.

The way I have been talking implies that tolerance levels are static unless the therapist intervenes. In fact tolerance levels vary according to stress levels. The more stressed a person is the lower their tolerance levels will be across a whole range of things. Helping clients to reduce the stress in their lives will usually increase tolerance levels. It is also possible to use specific procedures to increase tolerance levels to specific items. These are outside the scope of this book.

Foods, Food Phenolics & Food Additives

If you put something like an apple on CV6 and test TW21, and the muscle tests weak, it means that the client is allergic to that substance. The protocol discussed here offers a powerful way to fix allergies quickly.

It is usually important to check anything the client particularly likes, because allergy often equals addiction. If you ever hear someone say: 'I would be happy if I could live on X', there is a very good chance that they are allergic to whatever X is.

Also test anything the client particularly dislikes but still eats. Often small children instinctively dislike a food that is an allergen, but the parents insist the child eats it, because they believe that the food is good for the child, or they are concerned that the child will become a finicky eater.

Any food can be a problem. One of my sons was allergic to carrots, including organic carrots – they made him hyperactive. Interestingly he was fine on many of the foods and food additives commonly linked to hyperactivity.

Phenolic food compounds (also known as aromatic food compounds) occur naturally in all foods: they give the food colour and flavour and help to prevent premature decomposition. There has been research suggesting that some people who appear to have multiple allergies may be reacting to one of these compounds that is present in many different foods. Research (mainly by Abram Ber) also links particular phenolics to particular health problems.

For example, an allergy to apiol (found in beef, cheese, chocolate, milk, oranges, peas, black pepper, soybeans, tomatoes, almonds, carrot, celery, lettuce, parsley, walnut, bay leaf and lemon) has been linked to irregular menses, amenorrhea, menopausal flushing, breast tenderness, itching of skin, obesity, chronic fatigue and elbow pain. Checking and correcting food phenolics may enable you very simply to correct a wide range of allergens and improve a wide range of symptoms.

Many food additives cause problems. People can be allergic to artificial food colourings (e.g. tartrazine and sunset yellow), flavour enhancers (e.g. monosodium glutamate), artificial sweeteners (e.g. aspartame), preservatives (e.g. benzoic acid), and other chemicals that are added to our food by manufacturers.

When natural food colourings began to be used in processed foods, I was delighted. I had seen how many people were allergic to artificial food colourings, and the suffering they caused when this was not detected. I was very surprised and dismayed when I started testing these natural food colourings and found many clients reacted to them too, even though most of them were fine with the source material. For example the food colouring capsanthin (E160c) is derived from paprika, and I had clients who reacted to the food colouring but not to paprika itself. Initially this sort of a result mystified me till I learnt that solvents, such as methanol, hexane or acetone, were used in the extraction process to maximise the amount of the finished product. Minute traces of these solvents remain in the finished products, and sensitive clients react to them.

Sometimes a food that the client never eats shows as needing an allergy correction. See page 71 for one possible explanation for this.

See my book *Allergy A To Z* for more information on foods and food additives.

Inhalants, Contact Substances Etc.

Many practitioners concentrate on testing foods, but things people come into contact with and things they inhale are at least as important.

In our daily lives we breathe in dust, moulds, perfumes and at some times of the year pollens. We touch different types of wood, different fabrics, metals and ceramics. Any of these can be a problem for your clients. You can use this energy mismatch procedure to test and correct many of these problems.

In considering airborne substances it may be important to consider substances that originate a long way away. Volcanic dust, sand, pollens and pollution can be carried thousands of miles from their origin, so even though your client does not live near an active volcano or a desert, does not have a house in the country or does not live near a factory or an airport, you may still wish to test airborne substances that relate to these places.

Many chemicals are ubiquitous in the environment, so that in practice clients are often unaware of this sort of allergy, because they are unable to pinpoint a reaction that coincides with exposure.

Formaldehyde, for example, is one of the most common chemicals in the environment; it occurs in washing up liquid, cosmetics and personal care products; it gives paper 'wet strength', so is used in toilet paper and tissues; it is used in glue and so is found in chipboard and carpets; many non-crease, non-iron finishes applied to fabrics contain formaldehyde. This is not mentioned on the garment or bedding label: it may say 100% cotton, or 50% cotton and 50% polyester, but this does not mean that formaldehyde and other chemicals have not been used in the finishing.

Phthalates are chemicals that are found in plastics. They make plastics softer, but have been found to migrate into food or drink contained in the plastic, so some foods and many drinks are contaminated with phthalates. Your clients are exposed to these chemicals, and may need testing and correcting on them.

Benzene is given off when petrol/gas is put into cars. It is also used as an industrial solvent, in dyes, paints, adhesives and varnish removers, as well as drugs, and in the manufacture of nylon and other fabrics.

Triphenyl phosphate is a flame retardant added to many plastics such as TV's and computer monitors. When in use the appliance heats up and small amounts of this chemical vaporise into the air. This may affect people in an office even when they are not using a computer or similar equipment. Some people are aware that they react to electronic equipment, and put it down to the electromagnetic pollution, but triphenyl phosphate could be the problem, or certainly an additional factor.

These are a few examples. I hope they will help you realise that many of these chemicals are encountered in so many ways that it is vitally important to include them in your testing for at least some of your clients.

People encounter many things through their contact with other people. The client may not wear perfume, but will certainly be exposed to perfume worn by other people. A client who has no pets of their own may be exposed to cat hair on the clothes of friends. One of my sons would react with violent coughing to the cigarette smoke in people's hair and on their clothes, even though they had not smoked for several hours.

There are some allergens that are even less obvious at first sight, for example, a glaze used on crockery, or the stone used to build the client's house.

Nor should you be too rigid in your views about what sort of substances cause what sort of problems. I found that a small child, who only bed wet in summer, was allergic to some grass and flower pollens. One child with eczema was allergic to cotton.

Sometimes the client will know that they react in a certain room of the house or in a certain place, and you are unable to trace exactly what is causing the problem. In these circumstances I have found it is usually effective to get them to put a bowl of water in the place, leave it for about 24 hours and then bring it in for testing. The water will contain all sorts of airborne substances, and it may be possible to use the water for testing and correcting without knowing exactly what the problem is. I do not like doing this, but have used it as a last resort and found it very effective.

So, be prepared to test anything and everything. Do not decide that everyone is allergic to something, or no one is ever allergic to something else. Having said all that, I always advocate assuming that the situation is going to be simple, and testing obvious things first. If this does not resolve the problem, I widen the range of my testing.

My book *Allergy A To Z* has a comprehensive listing of what to test and why, and there is also more information on my web site and in the test kit information.

Dental Material

Dental treatment can be a real problem for a lot of people. A substantial number of people are allergic to dental anaesthetics and the materials used in modern dentistry.

The substance that most readily springs to mind is dental amalgam. People often refer to this as mercury, but in fact it is a mixture of different metals. Over half is mercury (in some older fillings that can be nearer three quarters), mixed with copper, tin, silver and zinc, so be sure either to test for amalgam or all the individual metals. Some people react to the plastics and porcelains that are now being increasingly used to replace amalgam.

It is ideal to test materials before they are used, but you may often be in the position of testing materials that are already in the mouth. This still works well and you can use the tapping procedure where appropriate to correct any problems.

Amino Acids

So far I have been looking at obvious reactions to foods and other allergens, but the energy mismatch procedure has implications for the way in which the body uses nutrients in foods.

The building blocks of protein are amino acids. When we eat protein the body dismantles it into its constituent parts in order for it to cross the gut wall. The body reassembles the amino acids into the proteins it needs.

Amino acids are involved in much that goes on in the body both structurally and functionally. They are used to make enzymes, some hormones, cell machinery, muscles, skin, hair, blood and antibodies. Some people react to one or more amino acids, and because of their importance and widespread use within the body this can have serious health implications.

You can learn more about amino acids in my book *Nutritional Testing For Kinesiologists And Dowsers.*

Minerals: Toxic And Beneficial

Minerals can be either beneficial or harmful. For example, lead, aluminium, mercury and cadmium are toxic minerals. Zinc, calcium and selenium are generally beneficial minerals. Copper is beneficial in very small quantities, but is harmful in larger quantities.

If an energy mismatch problem with toxic minerals is detected, it means that the energy system probably does not recognise the substance as toxic. This has several implications.

If the energy system does not recognise the energy pattern of a toxic mineral, the mineral is likely to be toxic at much lower levels than it would be for someone where the energy system did properly recognise the energy pattern. Using the tapping technique to correct an inability accurately to categorise a mineral as toxic will not stop a mineral being toxic, but will put the body in a better position to counteract the toxic effect of it.

If the energy pattern of a toxic mineral is not properly recognised, the body may not try to excrete it, but may prefer to store it, possibly treating it as a nutritious mineral that it is storing for use at a later date. This storing of a toxic mineral can cause all sorts of problems. Toxic minerals can be put in joints, in the brain, in the lungs, in the hair, the nails, and so on.

If the energy system does not properly recognise the energy pattern of a nutritious mineral, it will not make full use of it, because it may not try to absorb it fully. So, it is possible to have a situation where there is sufficient of a nutritious mineral in the diet, but the client is showing signs of a deficiency of that mineral, because the body is not absorbing the mineral properly. In some people the nutrition mineral that is not absorbed is not excreted, but is stored inappropriately, giving rise to a further set of symptoms relating to toxic overload. In other words you may have overt deficiency and excess symptoms within the same client. This can be very puzzling unless you understand about the energy mismatch concept. Using the energy mismatch tap where appropriate will fix both the deficiency and excess symptoms.

I had a good example of this with a client where testing revealed that her energy system did not recognize calcium properly and was putting the excess into her joints and causing arthritis. Her nails were brittle and weak, which is often a sign of calcium deficiency. I explained that she had symptoms of both excess and a deficiency of calcium and that this could be an inherited problem. She immediately told me that her mother had been in hospital recently for tests, and the diagnosis was abnormal levels of calcium around the heart. I never worked on the mother, but it seemed that she too had problems with calcium recognition, but her body dealt with it differently. In my clients case the excess was being put into the joints, and in her mother's case it was being put around the heart. Correcting the energy mismatch for my client resulted in a dramatic improvement in her arthritis, and her nails became much stronger too.

When the energy system has a problem recognising a nutritious mineral it is usually not appropriate to supplement with it immediately after completing the tap, but it may be important to do it later.

I believe there are two reasons for this. The first is that the body needs the experience of extracting the mineral from foods in the normal way, rather than being given a concentrated version of the nutrient.

The other reason, and this is probably more important, is that the energy system needs to extract the deposits that have been inappropriately stored and use these. If the client starts to take a supplement of the mineral, the body will almost certainly take what it needs from the supplement rather than using the stored mineral, thereby not correcting the problems of the stored excess. If I had supplemented my arthritic client with calcium after I had completed the tapping, her deficiency symptoms (brittle nails) would have probably improved, but her arthritis may not have improved, or only improved slightly. I normally use verbal questioning with muscle testing to check if it would be appropriate at any point to take the nutrient as a supplement. Even though I explain these concepts to clients, I have found that several have gone away and taken a supplement, so now I always tell them explicitly that they should not take a supplement for the energy mismatched substance (unless, of course, testing indicates that they should).

This problem of non-recognition and inappropriate storing casts an interesting light on basing the recommendation to use supplements on deficiency signs. If the reason for the deficiency sign is that the energy system does not recognise the energy pattern of the nutrient, giving more will probably reduce the deficiency signs, because the body is being "flooded" with the mineral, so more will get through. However, it is likely to increase the amount stored inappropriately. This may not have an immediate detrimental effect, but long term it is likely to lead to problems.

While teaching some practitioners about this problem of nutrient mis-categorisation, I remarked that white spots on the nails could be a sign of zinc deficiency, brought about by energy mismatch problems with zinc. One of the students had white spots on her nails, so she decided to check this out. Sure enough, testing showed that her body did not fully recognise zinc as a useful nutrient. She then corrected this. At a conference several months later she rushed up to me, held her finger nails in front of my face and said: "Look!" The top halves of her nails still had the white flecks, but the lower halves were completely free. Since completing the correction her nails were growing without the white flecks, showing that her body had learnt to recognize zinc and use it efficiently.

Regardless of whether you are testing toxic or nutritional minerals, the testing and correcting procedure is exactly the same as for allergies.

You can learn more about minerals in my book *Nutritional Testing For Kinesiologists And Dowsers*.

Vitamins

As with minerals energy systems can also fail to recognise vitamins. Water-soluble vitamins (such as the B and C vitamins) may be excreted when they are not properly recognised, although I am not totally certain of that. Fat-soluble vitamins, such as vitamin A and vitamin E are more likely to be stored and so cause symptoms of deficiency and excess.

In general it is not appropriate to supplement vitamins immediately after correcting an energy mismatch problem, for the same reasons that are discussed in the section on minerals.

You can learn more about vitamins in my book *Nutritional Testing For Kinesiologists And Dowsers.*

Essential Fatty Acid

Fatty acids are classified as essential or non-essential, depending on whether the body is able to synthesise them. The body is unable to produce essential fatty acids, such as linoleic acid and eicosapentaenoic acid, so must take them in via food or supplements. These essential fatty acids are important because the body uses them to make hormone-like substances called prostaglandins that are vital for good health. (See page 58 for more information on prostaglandins.) A fatty acid deficiency can lead to lack of energy and endurance, a poor immune system, high blood pressure, arthritis, dry skin and cracked nails. These symptoms can also occur when the amount of these essential nutrients is adequate in the diet, but the energy system does not recognise one or more of them properly.

Some people have problems with the conversion process changing essential fatty acids into prostaglandins within the body. Supplements of evening primrose oil and starflower oil (borage oil) supply GLA and so by-pass one of the steps in the conversion. These can be useful for people who have problems with the conversion process, but if the reason for the problem is that the energy system does not appropriately recognise the essential fatty acids themselves, the energy mismatch procedure can be used to correct this.

Supplements

Many clients will come to you already taking supplements. It is possible that these may be doing more harm than good. (See also *Nutritional Testing For Kinesiologists And Dowsers*.)

As well as the active ingredients in the supplement there are often several inactive ingredients. Coatings designed to mask the taste and make them easier to swallow include shellac (from a beetle), hydroxypropylmethyl cellulose and natural colourants (such as chlorophyll). Diluents, such as microcrystalline cellulose, dicalcium phosphate and soya bean oil, are used so that the active ingredients can be accurately dispersed in the tablets or capsule. Capsules are usually made from gelatine (from animals) and may contain glycerine to make the capsule softer and easier to swallow. Lubricants may be included to ensure that powders flow through machinery during manufacture. Lubricants include magnesium stearate, stearic acid, hydrogenated vegetable oil and silica in the form of silicon dioxide.

The client may be allergic to active or inactive ingredients in the supplement, giving rise to various symptoms. A client with psoriasis was doing really well, until she started taking cod liver oil for her arthritis. Her psoriasis flared up again, but I quickly identified and corrected the problem.

If the client is taking a mineral or vitamin supplement and the body does not recognise the energy pattern, there may be problems with inappropriate storage as explained in the section on minerals.

Bacteria And Viruses

The energy mismatch procedure is really useful for many clients with bacterial and viral problems. You test the energy patterns of these organisms in the same way as you test for the foods, minerals, etc.

Using the energy mismatch procedure where appropriate for people with an on-going infection can dramatically reduce the severity and length of the illness, and protect people against future exposure. I have had clients come in with sever colds or the beginning of flu and within less than half an hour they are symptom free. In fact many clients have commented that the symptoms start to disappear as the energy mismatch problem is corrected.

It can also be used where the energy system is still affected by an infection that happened in the past. One client, who developed psoriasis after having a sore throat caused by the streptococcus bacteria, responded very quickly to an energy mismatch correction on the bacteria. Within 10 days the psoriasis had become dramatically less red, sore and itchy.

Viruses

Viruses are the smallest known type of infective agent. Outside of living cells viruses are inert. They invade living cells, take them over and make copies of themselves. In general these are organisms that we do not want in the body, so it is vitally important that the energy system recognises them as harmful.

You may well find that you correct HIV and other alarming viruses. It could be because the client is currently infected with that virus, or it could be that it is necessary to do this, because the client is so susceptible to this life-threatening virus or bacteria that it is important to correct it in case they encounter it at some time in the future.

A good example of the efficacy of the energy mismatch procedure is in helping clients with cold sores. Cold sores are caused by the herpes simplex viruses (usually herpes simplex type 1), so check this out for anyone who suffers from cold sores. Using the vial you can test and correct the virus even when the client is not actively suffering from it. I have had almost 100% success at eradicating this distressing problem.

Bacteria

Bacteria are abundant in air, soil and water. Some are beneficial, some are harmful and some are thought to be harmless.

There are many bacteria that are harmful for humans. With the advent of antibiotic resistant strains this is in many ways a more pressing problem than viral infections.

It is easy to think solely of bacteria in relation to infection, food poisoning and respiratory problems, but bacteria (such as methicillin resistant staphylococcus aureus – MRSA) can have much wider implications than that. For example, streptococcus mutans is implicated in tooth decay, and helicobacter pylori in peptic ulcers.

If a harmful bacteria gets a weak response on muscle testing, this does not necessarily mean that the person has had a problem with that bacteria in the past. The test only shows that the person's system does not categorise the bacteria as harmful. However, if it is a common bacteria, it is likely that the person has been infected with the bacteria in the past and may have had a difficult time with it. It also may mean that in some way the physical body is still compromised by it. Using the tapping technique, if appropriate, will help to rid the energy system of this problem. Not recognising a bacteria as harmful also means that the person will be very susceptible to infection by that bacteria if they encounter it in the future.

Some bacteria are beneficial. There are bacteria in the gut that produce some B vitamins and vitamin K. Some bacteria provide a protective acid mantle on the skin. If these bacteria test weak on CV6, this is likely to mean that the body will be trying to rid itself of these beneficial bacteria. Correcting the problem allows the energy system to recognise these bacteria as helpful. Commensals are organisms that are often found on the human body, but do not appear to cause any harm. My own view on this is that commensals may well have some useful function, but as yet we do not know what that is. It seems unlikely that two organisms – human and bacteria – would be found constantly together without them having some symbiotic relationship, so it may be vitally important that the energy system categorises these commensals appropriately, so that that balance is maintained. In fact, there is now some research which is beginning to show that commensals may have a direct effect on the immune system, and may counter-balance more harmful bacteria, stopping them from growing out of hand.

It is important that the energy system recognises a bacteria appropriately. Otherwise it may encourage, or at least not actively discourage, the proliferation of harmful bacteria. It may try to destroy beneficial and commensal bacteria.

Sometimes bacteria or viruses will come up to be corrected that are not common now, and the person is unlikely ever to have been exposed to them. There can be several reasons that these come up. It may be that this is the closest energy pattern that you have to the one that the energy system wants.

Another possibility is that you are correcting an inherited miasm. This is a concept familiar to homeopaths, and refers to an inherited taint that has come down through the generations. The main miasms include syphilis, gonorrhoea and tuberculosis. Having an energy mismatch problem for T.B., syphilis, etc, does not necessarily indicate the presence of the disease, but may indicate a chronic tendency to manifest particular symptoms. For example, the person with a tubercular miasm is frequently nervous and tired; the person with the syphilitic miasm tends to be sulky, depressed and stupid, with problems with teeth and bones, etc. (Consult homeopathic texts for more information on this. *A Study Course In Homeopathy* by Phyllis Speight offers an excellent introduction to this fascinating topic.)

Fungus, Chlamydia, Rickettsia, Protozoa And Parasites

Fungus

Fungus are simple, parasitic life forms which cause illness by direct poisoning, toxic by-products, allergic reactions and/or colonisation of body tissues.

Various varieties of aspergilla cause severe respiratory symptoms. Athlete's foot is caused by a fungus, trichophyton rubrum. One important type of fungus is candida. When practitioners talk about candida they usually mean candida albicans, but other candida varieties (such as candida glabrata and candida krusei) are becoming an increasing problem so are well worth testing.

Chlamydia

Chlamydia are micro-organisms which are intermediate in size between viruses and bacteria. Like viruses they can only multiply by first invading the cells of another life-form. Otherwise they are more like bacteria and are susceptible to antibiotics.

Recent research on Chlamydia pneumoniae is very interesting. It has long been known that infection with this chlamydia can result in bronchitis pharyngitis, laryngitis, sinusitis and pneumonia. Recent studies have shown that the effects of this chlamydia can be even more worrying: people infected by it are 4.5 times more likely to have a stroke than matched controls who show no sign of having encountered it. Links have also been proposed with Alzheimer's disease, asthma, and some forms of arthritis. This is not a rare infection either: research has shown that by age 20 years, 50% of the population have evidence of past infection, and re-infection throughout life appears to be common. I do not know for certain if correcting an energy mismatch problem for this organism can prevent these long-term health problems, but I do believe it may.

Rickettsia

Rickettsia are a type of parasitic micro-organism. They resemble bacteria but are only able to replicate by invading the cells of another life form; rickettsia are parasites of ticks, lice, etc. These animals can transmit the rickettsia to humans via their bite or contaminated faeces. In my experience in the UK these are not a particular problem, but in other countries they seem to be a cause for concern.

Protozoa

Protozoa are the simplest, most primitive type of animal, consisting of a single cell. Giardia lamblia, E coli, Trichomonas vaginalis, and the Plasmodium family (malaria) are all protozoa, so this is an important energy mismatch category.

Parasites

Many therapists feel that parasites play an important part in illnesses, so you may want to test these. If there is an energy mismatch problem, this does not mean that the person has that parasite, although this will often be the case. Parasites have various life stages, and it is important to check the energy patterns of the different stages separately if possible. Roundworms (threadworms, pinworms and hookworms) have the simplest life cycle consisting of egg to larva to adult. Tapeworms have an additional stage: egg to larva to encased cyst to adult. Flukes have a different life cycle: egg to miricidia to redia to cercaria to metacercaria to adult.

Fungus, chlamydia, rickettsia, protozoa and parasites are corrected following exactly the same procedure as everything else.

Vaccinations

Personally I do not support wide-scale mass vaccination, but many of our clients will have been vaccinated before they come to us, or may decide to be vaccinated. Vaccinations can undoubtedly cause damage. The debate is about how much damage, and whether that is outweighed by the benefits of vaccination.

It is notable that when vaccines show up for the energy mismatch, clients will often remark that they had an adverse reaction to that vaccine, or have not felt well since they were vaccinated with that particular one. In either case correcting the energy mismatch problem can lead to greater health and well-being.

Clients may need corrections for vaccinations that were carried out many years ago, or they may be considering being vaccinated now. This most often comes up in relation to children, or when clients are having an exotic holiday. I try to provide clients with sufficient information that they can make an informed decision. If they decide to be vaccinated, you may be able to use the energy mismatch tap to counteract any adverse damage.

If the client is going to be vaccinated, I recommend that you test and correct the appropriate vials from the bacteria / virus kits and from the vaccination kit, both before and after vaccination.

If the client has decided not to be vaccinated, I test and correct the appropriate vials from the bacteria / virus kit. I also suggest the client reads *Vaccination Bible* by Lynne McTaggart or something similar for homeopathic alternatives etc.

Drugs: Medicinal And Recreational

Ideally we do not want our clients to be taking any medicinal or recreational drugs, but sometimes medicinal drugs are necessary either permanently or until the work necessary for the client to be able to live without the drug has been completed. In my experience many of the side effects of medication are because the energy system does not recognise the energy pattern of the drug properly. Using the tapping procedure where appropriate can allow the person to have the benefit of the drug without the side effects.

Clients can also be reacting to the non-active ingredients in tablets and capsules. See page 44 for more information on this.

It is always important to check for energy permission (see page 18) before undertaking the energy mismatch tapping technique, and it is particularly vital for medicinal drugs, because on rare occasions tapping for a drug may alter the dose of it that the client needs.

Do remember that in the UK, at least, it is illegal to tell a client to stop taking medication prescribed by their doctor.

Some people get addicted to recreational drugs more easily than others. This addiction usually shows up as an energy mismatch. Correcting this will help them fight the addiction more easily.

This test does not, of course, prove or disprove whether a client person has taken recreational drugs in the past or is taking them currently.

Drugs can remain in the system for many years. One client's energy system asked for a correction for a tranquilliser. I was surprised. When I told the client, he explained that many years ago he had had a serious nervous breakdown and had been in a mental hospital on high levels of medication. (He had not told me this when I took the case history.)

If you are helping someone to give up smoking, I suggest you check out nicotine and cotinine. In the body nicotine is broken down into cotinine. Cotinine is highly addictive and persists in the system longer than nicotine. Children and adults exposed to cigarette smoke in their environment may need to be checked for nicotine and cotinine too.

I have had some young children as clients who have needed corrections for recreational drugs that the mothers took before they realised that they were pregnant.

Hormones, Enzymes And Other Body Biochemicals

One of the most exciting and powerful ways of using the energy mismatch concept is with hormones and other body chemicals. The body produces many different chemicals in order to build and maintain itself. When things go wrong, ill health is the result.

Hormones are chemicals produced by the body in one organ that are transported around the body and have an effect elsewhere. They are one type of messenger molecules.

If the energy system fails to recognise the energy pattern of a hormone, it appears either to try to destroy it, or else it 'ignores' the message encoded within it. Either situation can result in severe health problems. Many clients have benefited from a treatment that involves an energy mismatch correction. It seems a particularly useful correction for people with thyroid, menstrual, blood sugar and weight problems.

An important group of hormones is those relating to reproduction and sexual characteristics. It is easy to have a simplistic view of the sex hormones, seeing some as being purely male and some as purely female, but women secrete testosterone, and men secrete a whole range of female hormones. In each case the quantity is smaller, but it is still there. For example, men produce prolactin, a hormone that promotes the secretion of milk from the mammary glands, but non-pregnant women produce 60% more, and pregnant women yet more still. Unfortunately it is difficult to find much information on the role of these sex hormones in the opposite sex.

Of course, not all hormone problems are caused by the energy system's inability to recognise the energy pattern of the hormone. Sometimes problems occur because a gland is damaged or malfunctioning for other reasons, and the problem will not show up using the energy mismatch test point, so the energy mismatch tap will not help in these situations.

Neurotransmitters

Neurotransmitters are chemicals that are released from nerve endings carrying the nerve impulse across the synaptic gap and onward to another nerve or a muscle cell or a glandular cell. This allows impulses to be passed rapidly from one cell to the next throughout the nervous system. Neurotransmitters include serotonin, acetylcholine, dopamine and GABA. Some neurotransmitters (e.g. noradrenaline) also function as hormones. The action of the neurtransmitor is either excitatory (stimulating) or inhibitory. Some neurotransmitters can be both, e.g. acetylcholine is excitatory at nerve/muscle junctions, but can be excitatory or inhibitory at nerve/nerve junctions.

Neuropeptides

Neurotransmitters consisting of 3-40 amino acids are known as neuropeptides. They are widespread in the central nervous system and the peripheral nervous system. They have both excitatory and inhibitory actions and work in a similar way to neurotransmitters. There are different types of neuropeptides: endorphins, methionine and leucine enkephalin, dynorphins, substance P, hypothalamic releasing and inhibiting hormones, and angiotensin II, all having different functions, and so can relate to a wide variety of problems.

Prostaglandins

Prostaglandins were first discovered in 1935 in seminal fluid and were assumed to be produced in the prostate, hence the name. Since then these hormone-like substances have been found to be continuously synthesised from essential fatty acids by most cells throughout the body. About 30 prostaglandins have been identified. Individual prostaglandins do not have a name, but are referred to as PG plus a letter and a number, e.g. PGD_1. They are generally quickly broken down, so they are short-acting substances. Unlike hormones they do not travel around the body, but do their work very close to the site of their production. Interestingly they can have completely different actions at different sites. For example, PGE_2, works in the reproductive system to stimulate contraction of the uterus, but in the respiratory system it widens airways. Some prostaglandins are involved with maintaining blood pressure, protecting against peptic ulcers, and controlling inflammation.

Enzymes

Enzymes are catalysts that speed specific reactions (usually millions or billions of times faster than without the enzyme). There are over 1000 different enzymes that we know about in the human body. There are likely to be many more that we do not know about. Enzymes are made from protein. A cell could theoretically produce a large range of different chemicals. The ones that are produced are determined by the presence of enzymes. If the energy system does not recognise the enzyme, it may try to break it down, or stop it in some other way from working effectively. Many enzymes require additional, non-protein, co-factors in order to be active. Zinc, manganese, potassium, sodium vitamins B1, B2 and nicotinamide are common co-factors. If the energy system has a problem recognising a co-factor, the enzyme may not be able to function properly, even when the enzyme itself is recognised appropriately.

Metabolic By-Products

The body is a chemical factory (as well as many other things), and these chemical actions produce metabolic by-products, such as urea, bilirubin, pyruvic acid and uric acid. If the energy system does not recognise these properly, it may not try to break down and excrete them, but instead seek to store them inappropriately, with resulting ill health for the client.

Although I have described separate categories of body biochemicals, in practice you may well end up correcting several in succession from different categories. For example, if your client has depression, you might want to test dopamine, beta endorphin, serotonin, anandamide and prostaglandin E_1, as well as the amino acid tryptophan.

If you have someone with blood sugar problems, there are lots of vials you would want to test including glycogen, insulin, glucagons, orexin B, salivary amylase, and the enzymes involved in glycolysis.

You can help people lose weight by checking and correcting leptin, somatastatin, neuoropeptide Y, CART, GLP_1 and all the digestive enzymes.

There are other body biochemicals that do not fit into these categories, such as the collagens, myoglobin, albumin and hydrochloric acid. These also can be relevant in the work you do for your clients. For a client with allergies and/or inflammation check out histamine, the complement factors and tumour necrosis factor alpha.

When clients are experiencing excessive pain, test anandamide, substance P, nociceptin and nocistatin. For gum problems check lysozyme and cathepsin C.

If you look at the test kit information on the Life-Work Potential web site or at the hard copy we provide free, you will see lots more possibilities.

Body Parts: Healthy And Diseased

Life-Work Potential sells test kits containing the patterns of both healthy and diseased body parts, and you may be able to obtain these from other suppliers. These can be used in the same way as any other vial. I do not recommend that these are used for diagnosis, but they can certainly be used to help people with a wide range of problems.

I have only recently had access to this type of sample, so I cannot be definitive about the way in which they work. It seems, however, that using healthy tissue vials may help to re-set the resonant frequency of that tissue or organ in the body. Using the tap for diseased tissues may help the body better to recognise the tissues as diseased, and take the necessary action to rectify that.

Sometimes you will find yourself using diseased tissue vials, but this does not necessarily mean that the client has that disease. It may be that the test kits you have do not contain a suitable example of a healthy tissue, and so the energy system chooses the diseased tissue. As with any substance, the energy system may be choosing the nearest match, because you do not have the exact vial available.

You may use a vial not because it is needed in its entirety, but because it contains a particular cell or cells. For example, there are various types of epithelium (the lining of organs etc.), so testing may indicate a particular organ, not because that organ is in any way defective, but because the sample contains a particular type of epithelium tissue.

A chronic disease vial may be indicated, not because the person has that disease but because they have the miasm / inherited taint represented by the chronic disease. (See page 48 for more on this.)

Body Substances

Using actual body substances in an energy mismatch is always a fascinating experience. The reason for using body substances is that the energy system is reacting to something in the body substance. The body substance contains something that the client is either having difficulty removing from the body or using inappropriately.

When you use body substances you will usually need to collect them in some way, so it is a good idea to keep tissues, scissors etc. in your treatment room. Also before testing a sample in a tissue, for example, test the tissue itself on CV6 to check that the client does not react to that. If they do, you will need either to correct that first, or else to use another receptacle.

There are lots of different body substances you can use.

Ear Wax

Ear wax often contains substances that are affecting the brain, or giving vertigo. Earwax can be collected using cotton buds (Q-tips), and then placed on CV6 for testing. Often the body will produce an excessive amount of ear wax when there is a substance in it that it is reacting to. Once the energy mismatch problem is corrected, the amount of earwax will usually quickly reduce to more normal levels, and other symptoms will improve or clear completely.

Nasal Secretions And Phlegm

Many people suffer from catarrh, runny noses and wheezy chests, so using phlegm and nasal secretions is a common procedure. The watery discharge produced by a hay fever sufferer is likely to contain some of the pollens that the person is reacting to. You may need to repeat the tapping throughout the season, because each time you use the discharge it will contain different pollens, depending on which plants are in flower at the time. Using nasal secretions when someone has a cold can often dramatically shorten the length of time the person has the symptoms.

Skin

Skin samples are frequently needed. They may be from apparently healthy skin, or from problem areas such as spots, skin tags, eczema or psoriasis. In skin diseases the body is often excreting substances inappropriately through the skin. This causes irritation and/or proliferation of skin cells. The easiest way to collect this is by putting a piece of sticky tape against the skin, pressing it down gently, and then peeling it off even more gently. This can then be put on CV6 for testing. I have had several male clients with psoriasis, who had a history of working with oils as engineers or mechanics. Testing showed that they did not recognise the energy pattern of these oils and appeared to be excreting some of this oil through the skin, causing or contributing to the psoriasis. One client had this problem even though it was some years since he had worked as an engineer. Correcting this using the energy mismatch procedure made a significant difference to their psoriasis.

Saliva

Saliva contains an amazing variety of substances. Medically saliva can be used to indicate HIV and drug abuse, and recent research has shown that it can be analysed for peptides and fatty acids related to cancer, Alzheimer, and heart disease. Analysis of saliva also shows up the early hormonal changes indicating pregnancy. Many childhood infections caused by bacteria and viruses can be confirmed clinically by analysing saliva. Saliva also contains some enzymes (e.g. lysozyme and salivary amylase /ptyalin). Although we are not conducting medical tests, this indicates the range of substances that can be found in saliva. I usually ask clients to spit on a tissue and place that on CV6.

Dental Plaque

Using dental floss to collect deposits from between the teeth may be particularly appropriate for someone with gum disease or heart problems. Researchers have found a link between periodontal disease and heart disease, but the exact mechanism is not yet understood. Periodontal disease in mothers has also been linked to pre-term, low birth weight babies.

Sweat

Sweat mainly consists of water, but there are also waste products, such as ammonia, urea, salts and sugar, as well as bacteria that enjoy a sweaty environment. You may be using sweat to correct one of these, or the sweat may contain other substances that the body is excreting through the sweat, and the tapping is correcting that.

Tears

Tears mainly consist of water. They also normally contain sodium chloride, a little mucus, antibodies, manganese and other minerals, and the enzyme lysozyme, which is anti-bacterial.

Vaginal Secretions

Vaginal secretions normally contain a range of hormones, but they may also contain other substances that the body is excreting inappropriately.

Semen

It may be necessary to test semen. Semen may contain many things, including protein fragments from food allergens. If a client is having difficulty conceiving, it is always worth testing her partner's semen on her.

Urine

There are many substances found in urine. Urea, chloride, sodium, potassium, phosphates, sulphates, creatine and some hormones `are normal constituents. Other metabolic substances (such as glucose, uric acid, proteins, albumin and bilirubin) may also be present indicating that something is wrong. In addition toxins are often excreted via the urine. Cotinine, the main breakdown product of nicotine, can be detected in the urine of smokers, and children and adults exposed to cigarette smoke. Other drugs and their break down products can also be found in the urine. Environmental toxins, such as organo-phosphates, may well be found in the urine. Other substances, such as titanium dioxide, which is used in tablets, capsules and mascara among other products, will be found in urine in clients exposed to them. If your client has an infection, microbes will also be found in the urine.

When I need a urine sample, I usually get the client to put a couple of drops onto some toilet paper and then wrap it in more toilet paper before putting it on CV6.

Nails And Hair

Minerals may be inappropriately deposited in the nails or hair. When this happens, they will often cause the hair or nails to be weak or break easily. It is easy to use a pair of scissors or nail clippers to collect these. Check if it needs to come from a particular part of the head or a particular nail.

Many clients report stronger hair and nails after these have been used in an energy mismatch procedure. This is probably because the minerals that are being placed inappropriately in the hair and nails are causing a disruption to their structure, so that they break easily. Once this has been corrected, the structure is no longer damaged and so the nails or hair can grow more strongly.

Stools / Faeces

I try and avoid using stools if possible, as these are not pleasant or easy to obtain, but on occasions they may be necessary. Normal stools contain a wide variety of substances including indigestible food residues, dead bacteria (including ones normally present in a healthy gut), dead cells shed from the lining of the intestine, and bile. Abnormal stools may also contain blood, pus, fat, parasites, heavy metals and harmful bacteria. The stools of clients who are lactose intolerant (but still consuming milk products) may well contain lactic acid and other short chain fatty acids that have been produced by the fermentation of lactose in the colon.

Breast Milk
Of course, this is not always a relevant body substance, but if a baby is being breastfed it should definitely be checked. One of my sons was highly allergic to eggs. If I ate eggs, the breast feed about eight hours later would result in him projectile vomiting across the room. It took me a while to realise what was the cause, because initially I did not understand that molecules from food I ate could enter breast milk.

Recent research has also shown that some environmental chemicals, such as bisphenol A, hexachlorobenzene, PCBs and PERC are present in breast milk, so a breast-fed baby could be reacting to these very toxic chemicals.

Blood
Blood contains a range of nutrients that will depend to some extent on what the client has recently eaten. It also contains the waste products urea and bilirubin. Fibrinogen involved in blood clotting, antibodies and complement factors involved in the body's defence system will also be present, as will a whole range of hormones being transported to their target sites. Cholesterol, homocysteine, chemicals and heavy metals will be in it too.

It is illegal to take blood in the UK unless you are medically qualified, and that includes intentionally pricking someone's finger. If you want to use blood you need to ask the clients to do it themselves unless you have the required qualifications. Using the fingertip blood testing equipment used by diabetics is the best way to obtain a sample.

The range of substances found in body samples is immense, and this is both an advantage and a disadvantage. It is an advantage because the substance you require may well be available in one or more body substances. The disadvantage is that along with the substance you want there may be many substances that the energy system does not want corrected at that time. It is of paramount importance that you ask for energy permission for the tap, as the body sample may contain other substances that the body is not ready to have corrected at that time. Fortunately many of these substances are also available via test kits for these occasions.

Sometimes it seems obvious which body sample to use. For example, if someone has a streaming cold, you may well use nasal secretions, whereas for someone with eczema you are likely to use a skin sample. However, it is important not to make any assumptions, but to test to find the appropriate one to use. (See more on this on page 73.)

In practice I often do not worry what I am correcting when I use a body sample, I just go ahead and correct it, although sometimes it is obvious, and sometimes it is interesting to know, so you can understand more about the process you are carrying out.

Flower & Gem Remedies, Homeopathics, Etc.

So far I have looked at substances taken into the body such as foods, food additives, pollens, dust, moulds, bacteria, viruses and drugs, and also at substances made by the body either for use (such as hormones, enzymes, neurotransmitters) or as part of the metabolic process, but there is a big additional category of substances: homeopathics, flower remedies, gem remedies and my earth energy remedies that you can use with this protocol.

So what does it mean if you put one of these energetic substances on CV6, hold TW21 and the muscle tests weak or unlocks? It means that the body does not recognise the energy pattern, so that the positive benefit of that energy is deficient in that person in some way.

You could, of course, take the remedy to rectify that problem, or you could tap it in (providing the tap will work and you have energy permission to do it).

Some people find this confusing. If you put an orange on CV6 and it tests weak, this means that the person should not eat the orange, but now I am saying that if a remedy tests weak they could take it.

This seems inconsistent, but it is not. There is a big difference between the orange and a flower remedy – one is a physical substance and the other is purely an energetic or vibrational pattern. One way of correcting an allergy to orange (which would show up on CV6) would be by giving a homeopathic version of the orange. If a substance tests weak on CV6, the client needs to avoid the substance in its physical manifestation till the problem is fixed, but the energetic manifestation can be tapped in or taken. This will correct an allergy and impart the positive qualities of the remedy.

It is interesting that sometimes people show up as reacting to a food that they never eat. It seems strange that the body wants it fixed, but remember everything has an energetic counterpart and it may be that the substance needs correcting for its vibrational qualities rather than its physical existence.

For example, in the Perelandra garden essences, celery is said to be the essence that restores balance to the immune system, cucumber is for periods of depression, and dill releases victimisation. So you could be doing what appears on the surface to be an allergy tap for cucumber, but it is not only that – it may also be helping the person to address the depression in their life. In fact you could be asked by the energy system to do a correction for cucumber even though the person does not eat cucumber, but needs the energy qualities to help them overcome depression. Any physical substance can be used as a vibrational remedy, by using it with the mismatch procedure.

The potency is usually unimportant when homeopathic remedies are used in the tapping procedure, although it may be vitally important when the remedy is taken.

There are repertories for homeopathic and flower remedies, but do not be surprised if sometimes a remedy comes up that appears to bear no relation to the description in the material medica. One of my sons had a severe cough, and testing indicated he needed a specific homeopathic remedy. I then read the information on the remedy, but it said nothing about any respiratory problems, so I did not give him the remedy. The next day his cough was worse, and again I tested for a remedy, and again I came up with the same remedy. As I had been testing without knowing what was in the bottles, this convinced me I should give him the remedy. Half an hour later he had stopped coughing. This was a long time ago, and I was much less experienced and confident in my muscle testing, so it taught me a valuable lesson. In this example I was giving him the remedy rather than using the tapping technique, but the same considerations apply.

The discussion on miasms on page 48 is also relevant to homeopathic remedies.

Deciding What To Test

By now you will have realised that there are many different things you can test, so how do you decide what to test? This can be done in several ways.

Sometimes the client has a good idea what is causing the problem, but sometimes they get it wrong or have no idea. I had one client who was convinced he was allergic to peanuts. Testing showed that it was the hops in the beer that he drank when he ate the peanuts that were the culprit.

You can use your understanding about what substances tend to cause what sort of problems. Symptoms that are worse at a particular time of day, or season, may suggest likely allergy culprits. Bacteria or hormones are linked to particular symptoms or illnesses, so you may want to test these when clients come to you with matching problems.

Allergy often equals addiction, so ask your client if there is anything they particularly like to eat or drink, and make sure you test it. Ask your client if there are any common smells that most people do not like, but they like, and test those. A client who likes the smell of creosote or petrol (gasoline) is likely to be allergic to the substance. There is a lot more information about this in my book *Allergy A To Z.*

You could just test everything that you have available, but this is likely to be an extremely long and inefficient process.

Sometimes intuition, or experience, or information from your client, will suggest where to start, but it is also important to have a systematic and reliable method for when these fail or are not appropriate. Verbal questioning with muscle testing can quickly allow you to narrow down the options. Typical questions include:

> 'Is the next thing we correct something the client has brought with them?'
>
> 'For the next correction are we looking for something I have in my office?'
>
> 'Are we now looking for something from one of the test kits I have?
>
> Do we need a body substance next?'

Do remember that the energy system may want several substances corrected in a session, but in a particular order, so that your questioning needs to be focussed on the next substance to correct. My book *Verbal Questioning Skills For Kinesiologists* will give you help and guidance on how to do this sort of questioning quickly and accurately.

You can, of course, use a mixture of the different approaches both in different sessions and within sessions. The important thing is that you keep an open-mind about what to test, and then test as objectively as possible.

Managing The Session

You are unlikely to want only to correct one substance, so how do you manage the session.

Once you have found and corrected the first substance, you need to establish if it is appropriate to do more. I usually do this by asking the verbal question:

> "Do we have energy permission to continue testing and correcting more things?"

A strong/locked muscle response means that yes, you do. If you get a weak/unlocked response, do not continue. This does not, of course, mean that you cannot correct more in the future. You may even be able to do more in this session after you have done some other work. In general though the energy system is very happy to have quite a few of these corrections done in a session. Once you have corrected the second item, you ask the question again, and, providing you get a strong muscle response, you continue with another item.

There may come a time when you want to stop, and it is important to make sure that it is appropriate to do so. Again I establish it using verbal questioning and muscle testing. This time the question is:

"Do we have energy permission to stop?"

A strong/locked response means that you do. If you get an unlocked response, it is vitally important to continue. It may be that you need to use the energy mismatch procedure for one or more additional items, or it may be that some other type of work is needed.

Appendix 1: The Full Protocol

1. Complete the thymus tap (page 7)
2. Check the energy system is balanced (page 9) and, if you wish, run your normal pre-checks
3. Establish which substance you are going to test (page 73)
4. Test the substance (page 14)
5. Check that the energy mismatch procedure will work (page 17)
6. Check you have permission to correct the problem (page 18)
7. Carry out the tap (page 20)
8. Recheck the energy mismatch point (page 21)
9. Check that the correction is now robust (page 22)
10. If you wish to do more, check that is appropriate to continue (page 75). If "yes", go back to step 2
11. If you wish to stop, check that it is appropriate to stop (page 76)

Appendix 2: Containers Used In Testing

Substances for testing may be in a variety of containers. For example, clients may bring food wrapped in plastic or aluminium, or in plastic storage boxes. Bottled water, supplements and homeopathic remedies may come in plastic containers. Juice cartons are sometimes lined with aluminium, and some chocolate is sold wrapped in it.

In general I do not find that I get accurate results testing through metals. The metal seems to 'block' the energy pattern of the substance, so you will need to remove things from tins or aluminium packaging before testing.

Plastic can also be a problem for two very different reasons. Some people are allergic to plastic so would test weak on anything contained in plastic. (Occasionally you will find some people who are only allergic to some types of plastic.) If you want to test things through plastic, you can check first that the client is not allergic to it.

If the client is allergic to plastic, you have two options:

1. Correct the plastic allergy first (providing you get energy permission to do so)
2. Decant everything into glass, paper, etc.

An equally important issue is that there is quite a large group of people who do not test well through plastic: any substance contained in the plastic will test as being fine, even when it is a problem. Interestingly these people are usually very sensitive to electro-magnetic disturbances. This can be corrected temporarily by using a hairdrier to degausse the body.

Degaussing involves a simple but seemingly odd procedure where a small electric motor is passed briefly over the whole of the body. A hairdryer provides a suitable motor. You use the side of the hairdryer moving the motor (not the hot air outlet) gently and slowly over the body. Make sure you do the whole body, including under the feet. The whole procedure only takes a couple of minutes. After that you should be able to test successfully through plastic for the rest of that session, although you will probably need to degausse the client again in future sessions, unless you correct the underlying problem with other techniques.

Most clients who need this in order to be tested properly will also benefit from degaussing on a regular basis, often once a week. It takes only a few minutes and people often report feeling more 'awake' when they start doing it regularly. They are also generally less susceptible to geopathic stress and electro-magnetic pollution. Problems with static electric shocks seem to disappear and people often become much less 'addicted' to television and video games.

Whatever containers you are using, you need to watch out for a client reacting to everything in a particular type of container. If this occurs, you will need to test the container on its own. If it is a problem, either correct that before continuing, or else put those things into a different type of container.

Appendix 3: Turning Off Allergic Reactions

The tapping technique can be used to turn off allergic reactions while they are happening, so you can teach clients this as a simple but highly effective self-help technique. The sooner the client becomes aware of a problem and the quicker the tapping is started the better the result will be. The client taps the same points as are used for the tapping correction (see page 21), but they do not put a substance on CV6. This does not correct the allergy permanently, but it does temporarily turn off the allergic reaction.

This can even be done when the client is aware of their normal allergy symptoms developing, but is not aware of what is causing the problem. They just tap the points, and 'magically' their allergy symptoms usually disappear or at least lessen.

Long term, of course, you want to correct all the allergies so that the client does not experience any problems, but teaching them this first-aid measure can be very useful in the early days of treatment for complex cases.